Brain Trauma and a Road to Recovery

There Is Hope

Steve Flores

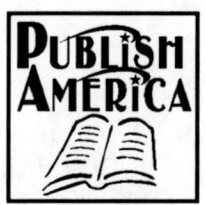

PublishAmerica
Baltimore

First printing

PublishAmerica has allowed this work to remain exactly as the author intended, verbatim, without editorial input.

ISBN: 1-60813-981-6
PUBLISHED BY PUBLISHAMERICA, LLLP
www.publishamerica.com
Baltimore

Printed in the United States of America

Thank you to my family and friends for their continued love and support throughout the years. I would like to especially thank Paul who is both my father and my best friend. His invaluable love, dedication, acceptance, and unending support enabled my success and words cannot adequately express my undying gratitude.

Introduction

"I'm about to die!" is the last thing I remember when I was about three inches from hitting the pavement.

I landed on my front right foot, falling forward with my arms out and eventually landing on my face. I broke my right foot, 8 ribs, my left shoulder, my chin and the tip of my right elbow. Also broken was my maxilla (the area behind a person's top lip), both jaw joints, my nose, and the surrounding area were all crushed. I also shattered my left cheekbone and half of my left eye socket. Additionally, I significantly injured my back.

As soon as my head hit the ground I was immediately in a coma. Months after recovering, a police officer from the scene of the accident told me that he heard my heart stop beating and he was sure that I had died.

This book is intended to help families with loved ones who have brain trauma whether it is a closed head injury, brain surgery or a stroke and to help the injured person understand what happens when there is severe brain trauma. Also the following chapters describe the stages that are experienced after a head injury, to let them know about the recovery process, and to inform them that there is hope.

I am not a doctor, but this is my experience as a survivor of serious brain trauma. The following chapters describe how I went from almost dying on March 21, 1999, at the age of 30, to waking up completely mentally and physically disabled, and deformed facially, to my recovery, and how I eventually found success and happiness in all aspects of my life.

Immediately After the Accident

The initial shock of the phone call informing the family that a loved one has been in an accident is horrific. In my case, the stress for my dad, mom, sister, extended family and friends was huge, but I am grateful that I did not have a spouse or children because it would have been even worse.

Months after coming out of the coma, I read the emails that my mother sent to loved ones. Below are the heartbreaking emails in chronological order.

1. "Steve was in a very bad car accident and he will most likely not be with us tomorrow morning."
2. "Steve had a rough night and we almost lost him a number of times, but somehow he made it through the night."
3. "The doctors are hoping that someday Steve will come out of the coma some day, but most likely he will be in a coma or in a 'vegetative state' for the rest of his life."
4. "They spent 4 hours in surgery to remove bone fragments that could cause further injury and so they could put him on a ventilator, but they said that they could not do all of the facial surgery needed at this point because Steve would die in the operating room because the surgery would be too much additional trauma."

The fourth email above was sent only 12 hours after the accident and I did not have my second facial surgery until 5 days later which took 11 hours.

With my grave prognosis and uncertain future, my family was terrified, had endless questions, and was in the dark. Eventually, they found a doctor to help answer their questions named Dr. Jeffrey Dombrowski (my maxillofacial surgeon). Dr. Dombrowski came to my families rescue and with his selfless attitude he helped my family while I was in a coma and for months afterwards.

At a point like this, family and friends need doctors, nurses, rehabilitation experts, counselors, and other experts to inform the family of what is and what will go on as well as prayers or good thoughts which help them immensely. My advice is to keep asking questions and, if you don't find someone with answers, keep looking. There will be someone who will take time to answer your questions.

Memories and Finding an Advocate

Many questions are frequently asked and are probably on the mind of the family members and friends of someone with brain trauma. Some of these questions include "Did you see a bright light and a tunnel?", "what was it like being in a coma?", and "what do you remember?"

An individual's personal beliefs about what happens when you die are important because they help determine what they will experience. If a person believes that there is a bright light and a tunnel, then that is most likely what that person will experience. Although I must have had some brief initial thoughts, I do not remember any of them.

It is speculative on my part, but many doctors I have spoken with have agreed with the following: although the time that it takes for the trauma and brain swelling to render a person in a coma varies, there is some amount of time for this transition to occur. This is when some people might "see a bright light at the end of a tunnel."

The time that it takes to come out of a coma varies from person to person. For more information do an internet search for Rancho Coma Scale. Each brain injury is different. In my case, I was in a coma for 26 days and there are only three things that I remember.

The first memory I have of being injured took place in what is best described as the Civil War era. I was in a canoe, injured, and my sister was taking care of me, explaining that I was injured and that things were going to be okay.

Interestingly, my sister was at my bedside for the first 10 days or so immediately after my accident, so I believe that this is the time of this memory. The important thing to note is that, although a person with a head injury might not respond, some things that are said or done are heard at times. Talking to or doing something for someone in a coma is never a waste of time because, at a minimum, you are stimulating the injured person's brain.

In my second dream-like memory, I was in a wheelchair at a hospital and can remember that I was being transferred from one location to another, feeling confused and not being able to help myself or able to get up. I suppose this was after I was taken off the ventilator and starting to come out of the coma while someone on the medical staff was taking me somewhere for tests.

The third thing that I remember is when I was coming out of a coma, there was a nurse chastising me for going to the bathroom in my bed. Although the vast amount of people in the medical field are compassionate and caring, this nurse held my legs together with one hand like the way people do when changing a baby's diapers and told me that if I wanted "to be treated like an adult I would have to start acting like an adult."

The lesson from my third memory is that family and friends need to be an advocate for the injured person. Let me reiterate that most people in the medical industry care and care a lot. But, for those who either are having a bad day or treat their position like any other job, you need to remember that meeting with the nurses and doctors is important so they know that someone is watching.

Coming Out of the Coma

Coming out of a coma is seldom accomplished in a short amount of time and knowing what to expect is important. It took me a few days to come out of the coma. The first few days that I began to remember significant events the way that I believe they actually occurred are important because they are common among most head trauma survivors.

After the ventilator tube was removed from my left nostril, I still had a feeding tube in my right nostril, my jaw was wired shut, and I had a tracheotomy, which made it so I could not speak. I could only read things 3 inches from my face because my brain injury was in the back of my brain (the occipital lobe), which is the vision center for your brain. Gesturing and writing everything that I wanted to say was very frustrating.

It is not unusual when a person is on a ventilator for them to get pneumonia. I had pneumonia and went from 215 pounds to 155 pounds, but the doctors said that being heavy helped me survive.

Whether the brain trauma is from a head injury, stroke, or surgical procedure, the hallmarks that are frequently experienced are confusion, depression, and anxiety.

Initially, my thoughts were scattered and incorrect. I thought that my accident happened while going from church-to-church looking at Easter scenes. Easter actually occurred in 1999 almost 3 weeks after my car accident, so this was not realistic.

Several days passed before I understood and believed how the accident actually happened. My short-term memory was poor at best, which made my confusion greater.

My mood for the first few weeks was most often upbeat and friendly to the point of not being realistic with my circumstances. I was flirtatious and I was grabbing nurses inappropriately. Later, a rehabilitation counselor informed me that this is not uncommon.

Part of my anxiety was caused by withdrawal affects from no longer being on strong pain medication. I was not told about the withdrawal and this is important for the injured person to know so they can understand why they are having anxiety. I refused any strength of pain medicine as soon as I was conscious in part because of not being in touch with reality and very correctly understanding that if I was sedated I would not be able to recover as fast or, most likely, ever.

The next shock after an accident like this is the first time you see your face. My face was disfigured and, even though I was told that things could be fixed, it was a scary reality check.

No matter if a family member or friend just dropped by briefly or for a longer period of time, this is very important for anyone in the hospital. Not only does a patient need reassurance and the feeling of being loved, but the survivor also wants to be kept company because being in a hospital is incredibly boring.

It was exceptionally boring because the hospital I was in had only three TV channels. What made it worse were the only things that were on was the Columbine High School shooting and Wayne Gretski retiring.

Rebuilding My Life

The severity and location of the brain trauma determines the struggle ahead. Doctors have confirmed my belief that if an area of a brain is damaged and not destroyed, it can be rebuilt.

Fortunately, my brain was damaged in a number of areas, but no areas were destroyed. Although I could communicate very shortly after I cam out of the coma, I would have to relearn almost everything.

Rebuilding your life is tough, but it also gives you the opportunity to build the exact life that you want for yourself. Many people, me included before the accident, are not happy with all aspects of their life, but feel it is impossible to drastically change their life. With a brain injury like mine, you have no other option but to make drastic changes. If you can achieve your goals, it is amazing to be able to have the exact life that you want.

Performing Basic Functions

The recovery process began and going home was the first major goal. The first two items I needed to accomplish were to be able to go to the bathroom on my own and to be able to eat enough calories to heal and stay healthy.

One motivating factor to be able to go to the bathroom was to get rid of the catheter. They are uncomfortable and painful when your leg or something else tugs on it. The only way to be able to go the bathroom on your own comes through trial and error, with and without the catheter in. There are some accidents and it is embarrassing, but the feeling of getting back to being able to perform normal daily items helps a person get through this challenge.

The next step was to be able to feed myself and eliminate the feeding tube in my nose. The doctors said that, until I stopped drooling on myself, they would not take the feeding tube out.

It took me five days or so to stop drooling. I was motivated to be able to eat and recover, but I also wanted the feeding tube out because I could not drink water and I felt incredibly thirsty at times. The nurses can actually adjust your IV and, within minutes, the feeling of being thirsty goes away, but you still want to be able to satiate that craving immediately.

Once the feeding tube was removed, I learned that I could not drink thin liquids, which was disappointing and frustrating. The reason for this is because while a person is in a coma the epiglottis (what seals off the windpipe when eating and drinking) is not exercised and loses strength. So until it re-strengthens thin liquids can go into your lungs which can cause pneumonia.

My jaw was wired shut so my diet consisted of custard style yogurt, pudding, mashed potatoes, and applesauce. It was kind of humiliating because I knew that I looked like an infant smashing food into my mouth with a significant amount of the food ending up on my face.

The doctors said that one requirement was that I had to be able to eat 2500 calories a day. The reason for the large amount was that my body needed more calories to be able to heal. After a few days of eating on my own, I was able to eat the required amount of calories.

Cognitive Requirements to Leave the Hospital

To be able to leave the hospital, I had to pass some cognitive tests. I had already accomplished being able to go to the bathroom by myself and being able to eat enough calories.

The rehabilitation therapist and I argued (via me writing) the extent of my brain injury. I thought that I was fine, I was frustrated and little pissed off on his insistence that I had the two scary words; "brain damage."

After any serious head trauma, there are batteries of cognitive tests that are administered to determine what areas of the brain are injured or destroyed. Though I was able to score high enough on the tests that doctors and therapists could not force me to go to a rehabilitation floor, it would still take seven and a half years to fully recover.

As I have seen with friends who have had head injuries or other brain trauma, it is not unusual for the person to think that they are fine and being held without just cause. It also seems common that people just want to go home, as I did. Numerous things were not right with my thinking. The following are just a few examples:

Although I could remember things that happened before the accident, I could not recall people's names. If the television were on, I would think to myself, "oh, oh, I know that persons name," but I could not remember even the most popular celebrities like Eddie Murphy or Dan Rather.

Another example is how I would not use the correct words in sentences and wouldn't recognize my mistakes. I would often use a word that sounded similar, For instance, I would say, "they injected my face with sterile to help reduce the swelling," when I meant to use the word "steroids" instead of the word "sterile."

My ability to do math in my head was gone and also was some reasoning ability. I would understand that if I did A, then B would happen, but I could not see other issues that might occur. For example, if someone told me to "put on my seatbelt because it is the law," I would not recognize that it also would help me avoid injuries if I was in an accident.

There are endless other examples, but the point is that there may be a wide range of items that a person with brain trauma will have problems with, some that they recognize and are frustrated with, and some that they do not even recognize. Family and friends need to be understanding and encouraging.

Other Issues Before Leaving Hospital

Brain trauma can have a big impact on your equilibrium. Mine was best described as being stumbling drunk. It took three rehabilitation people to help me walk. One would stand behind me with a leather belt under my armpits and the other two would be on either side holding me up.

After being on a ventilator for so long and still having some mild pneumonia, making it down the 40-foot hallway and back was tough. The distances slowly increased, but after my once or twice a day walk, I was exhausted.

My ability to walk and my equilibrium made some huge improvements over the next two weeks. I was able to walk alone, albeit holding the wall because I refused to use a walker. Around this, time the rehabilitation person took me to a kitchen to see if I could get something out of a cabinet and put it in the microwave. This might sound simple, but depending on the location and severity of the brain trauma it is a big deal because you can't go home until you can take care of yourself. I was able to pass this test, so another issue was taken care of.

At this point I was able to go to the bathroom on my own, eat the required amount of calories, passed the cognitive evaluation, walk, and get around the kitchen somewhat. Now the final hurdle before leaving the hospital was being able to breathe with the tracheotomy tube shut. In addition to me being able to go home, this would also allow me to be able to speak.

A nurse put in a temporary tracheotomy tube that allowed me to practice breathing with the tube closed. From being on a ventilator for an extended period of time, my diaphragm had become very weak and the pneumonia made this even worse. I remember the first time I closed the tube, I was laboring for air and I could keep it closed for only about 15 seconds before I had to open it again. I tried a couple more times and got up to about 25 seconds.

At this point, I was frustrated and scared. I even started to accept the fact that I would have a tracheotomy for the rest of my life and that I would just communicate with the world through writing.

The next time I saw the trauma surgeon, I explained how I felt and he suggested to "try standing up because you broke bunches of ribs!" This was encouraging because this meant that I might be able to get rid of the tracheotomy. It was also distressing that I had to experience intense moments of fear and depression because I was not told that I had broken a number of ribs.

Within three days, I was able to cap the tracheotomy tube full time and able to walk with it capped. Before I was released, the doctors wanted to see if I was going to be able to drink thin liquids. The test showed that thin liquids still were going into my lungs which was a big disappointment because this meant that I could not drink water.

Subsequently, the nurse showed me a product called Thicken, a powder that you could put in any liquid to make the liquid it thicker. Very quickly, I found that a lot of things aren't the same thickened, like chunky milk.

Going Home and the First Few Days

Forty-two days later, my doctor came in and said that I was going home! Although I would still have my tracheotomy tube and jaw wired shut, I did not care because I was leaving the hospital! I spent the next two hours with my doctors and nurses to complete the required exit information and it felt like the two hours lasted forever.

My mother came to the hospital to take me home. Being outside of the hospital was a huge a relief and it was also amazing to see the world again. Because my brain injury occurred in the back of my brain, which is a person's vision center, the sun and bright lights hurt my eyes. Luckily, this was easily fixed with sunglasses.

Since I had not been home in six weeks and because of the special diet (the same as in the hospital: custard style yogurt, pudding, mashed potatoes, and smoothie drinks) I would be on for the next eight weeks, we went to the grocery store. Sounded great, but this would be the first time that I was around people who did not know me.

I hobbled around the grocery store with my mom, got the five things that I would be eating for the next eight weeks, and went to the checkout. Everything seemed good, but the first child that I encountered was terrified and almost started crying when he saw me because my face was so badly disfigured.

I tried to console the child by telling them that I was in a car accident and that everything would be okay, but to no avail. Even though it appeared that I handled this well and was not bothered, it was the first time that I realized how bad I looked.

For most people, this amount of activity is a small part of a regular day. But for me, by the time I got home, I was exhausted and went to sleep.

In the morning, the medical supply company came over to drop off the items the doctor had recommended: morphine drip, walker, cane, suction machine to clean out my tracheotomy tube, portable toilet, and a chair so I could sit in the shower. I refused all, but the cane and the shower chair.

About three days out of the hospital, my mother came over to help me go through a pile of bills. To write ten checks probably took an hour and a half because of my confusion. At that time, I recognized that this everyday kind of task was very difficult for me, took a lot longer than it used to, and was another source of frustration.

Over the next week, I slept around twenty hours a day. I would get up only to go to the bathroom, eat, go to a doctor's appointment (I had four or five appointments a week early on) and an hour of cable television was the highlight of my day.

Either way, being home was better than being in the hospital. Even though I recognized that simple things were difficult, I was still unrealistic thinking that I would recover mentally and emotionally, as well as my face being fixed, in less than six months.

Short-Term Recovery

My living environment was not favorable for my recovery. My high school friends living in town and the friends that I had made after college had been going in a different direction than what I wanted before the accident, but I had not broken away.

Additionally, I was going to have to recover on my own. My roommate and people who were supposed friends, were not of much help. My mother lived in town, but she worked and the rest of my family lived in other states.

I understand that the grave forecast for my future was part of me recovering on my own. The doctors and my family hoped that I would be able to live alone and maybe find a part time job someday. My family, friends, and doctors also knew that the facial reconstruction was going to take a lot longer than the six months that I thought.

Today, I recognize that in most situations, it is pretty much impossible to ask someone to stop working when they need the money, drop their life, and embark on what doctors thought was going to be an impossible task of helping me rebuild my life from the bottom up with so much brain trauma. I am not bitter at all, but I recognize that part of being single is that if you are going to recover, you are most likely going to have to do it on your own.

For the first two weeks I was home from the hospital, a nurse would come over to help me clean around my tracheotomy and help with a couple of household items. It was comforting to know that she was there to help and that, if I needed more help, she could come more frequently.

About a week after I got out of the hospital, I went to a mental rehabilitation specialist for a couple of weeks and learned an important lesson: the things that you are not good at are the things that you need to try the most. It was extremely frustrating to not be able to do things that once came easily because I did remember how simple those things used to be for me to do.

I needed to get rid of this attitude because it did not matter the way that it used to be, but instead, the way that it was currently. I was motivated to get better, but my inability to do simple things was still a major source for my depression.

Shortly afterwards, I bought some books that elementary kids read for mathematics (addition, subtraction, multiplication, division and fractions), books on grammar, a dictionary to carry in my pocket everywhere I went, logic books, crossword puzzles, and anything else that I could find to "workout" my brain.

It was a big reality check once I started doing problems and reading the books. I would think to myself and say to my father, "I am totaled, my life is over, and I am never going to do anything or be anyone." My father is a very levelheaded and caring. He consoled me and encouraged me to continue to move forward and to look back every couple of weeks and celebrate the progress and achievements that I had made. Even at the bottom and looking up, this kind of compassion, motivation and direction made sense and kept me moving forward.

Another item that was a source of frustration was that my right eye would not shut because of nerve damage from crushing my right jaw joint. My maxillofacial doctor said to wait for a couple of months to see if the nerve was injured and would recover or if I needed to have microsurgery to fix it.

Within about a month, I could close my which was exciting for me. Walking around with your eye taped shut or your eye pegged open is embarrassing. Although eventually I could close my eye, I still can only move my right eyebrow slightly, but it is not noticeable so I really do not think about it very often.

For the first three weeks, I did not drive because of confusion, my vision was not very good, and it was too exhausting. The first time I drove to the grocery store about a mile a way and back was grueling and looking back now, I realize that I was not ready to drive. Again, I thought that I could drive because I had been driving for years and it was simple before the accident, but this was not the case after the brain injury.

Midrange Issues and Challenges

The first month out of the hospital had passed by with some successes and some frustration, but there was a lot of work ahead. The following are some of the midrange issues and challenges that occurred over the next 18 months. There were many, but I have noted only some because not all of my issues and challenges will be experienced by someone else with a brain injury. The important part of the below challenges is the way that I handled them and they will give you good ideas on how to handle challenges in general.

First, something positive, the big day had arrived. Fourteen weeks from the day of my accident, my jaw was going to be unwired. I was ecstatic. This meant that I could eat and my tracheotomy tube would finally be removed; well, at least that's what I thought.

I was put under partial sedation so the arch bars and wires could be removed, but when I woke up I found that I could not open my mouth more than a third of an inch. At first I thought eating normal food with a fork would happen in a week, but, again, this was not going to be the case at all.

The muscles in my jaw had atrophied (essentially shrank) so the way to get my mouth to open again was to stretch the muscles. This was accomplished by placing as large of a stack of tongue depressors between my teeth and then sliding another one in to stretch my mouth open. To say the least, this was extremely painful and it took four weeks before I could open my mouth normally; painful, but another victory on the road to recovery.

Even after the four weeks, my jaw was incredibly sore. It actually took nine months before I was able to chew a thin steak. The good news is that right after my jaw was unwired; I did not have to eat only food that I could smash through my teeth.

The next issue was my equilibrium, which was still poor at best. One example of the problem of balancing was when I was in the restroom at a movie theater and a man came in and was looking at me because I was swaying back and forth. I told him, "I am not drunk; I was in a car accident," this was embarrassing.

With my equilibrium problems, there was really no cure except time. Still today, ten years later, if you walk next to me for about 100 yards, I will kind of tilt into you. At this point in my life, I look at this as a minor issue and, comparatively, it is not a big deal.

An interesting memory issue was when I went to the mall; I would forget where I parked my car. Even eighteen months after the accident, I still remember spending three hours looking for my car in a mall parking lot. This is something that has improved, but I still have problems.

To accommodate this issue now, I usually go to the same mall and park in front of the same store. If I am at a new mall, I always park by the food court. Also, having a car alarm helps because even when I get to the area where I parked, I still often do not remember what spot I parked in. So turning the alarm on helps solve this problem.

A second memory issue was when I was traveling. Even four years later, I once showed up to the airport ready to go, but my flight was actually the following day. In addition, I would forget to bring very important things like my medicine or cell phone.

Still today, ten years later, I have some problems with traveling. To compensate, I mark the date on my calendar, send an email to myself with the itinerary, and before I leave, I check the dates and times a number of times. As for forgetting items, I write a checklist, pack the night before, go through the list that night, and go through the list again before I leave. Forgetting medicine can be a disaster, so I always have one bottle in my luggage, one in my carryon bag, and sometimes I even ship one to my destination.

Still today, my directional sense is not very good. However, right after the accident it was terrible. I could get lost for long periods of time and I would often travel in the wrong direction for 20 or 30 miles before I would recognize this and eventually have to turn around. Today, I do not use a GPS because, again, practicing what you are not good at is the only way to learn and improve.

A further difficulty I experienced was that my mind was still not clear six months after the accident. Unfortunately, a girl took financial advantage of me. It is better stated that I was mentally disabled at that point and I was not able to understand people's intentions. This is something that I assume happens on a regular basis and the only way to avoid this is to be around people that you know and have your family or friends help direct you.

Another issue I had was being scalded in the shower because I did not understand which way to turn the water on in the shower. Obviously, turning on the water was something that I had done for decades, but my confusion really was this bad. My solution here was turning the hot water heater down.

Finally, my prescription coverage ran out and my medicine was about $700 per month. There are a number of things a person can do in this situation; the first is to ask your doctor if they have samples because they usually do. Next, there are pharmacy chains that you can pay a relatively small fee and get 10 to 20% off on your prescriptions.

Third, many pharmaceutical companies have programs that if you earn less than a particular amount of money annually you can get the medicine at discounted prices. There are also non-profit groups that help people who are uninsured or underinsured get the medicine that they need. Finally, if you meet the requirements for Medicaid, you should apply because Medicaid makes your prescriptions very inexpensive.

Surgeries

Having broken, crushed, or shattered every area of my face created a need for numerous surgeries and procedures. As mentioned before, I thought that it would take less than a year, but I was not in touch with the severity of my facial injuries and the time frame that I was thinking of was simply unrealistic.

Below is a partial list of the surgeries and procedures that I had:

• 4 hours of initial surgery immediately after the accident to fix areas of my face enough so further damage would not occur and so I could be put on a ventilator
• 11 hours of facial surgery 5 days after my accident. An interesting note is that the doctor took a large piece of my jaw that had broken off and used it to create a floor for my left eye socket. Bone breaks like slate in layers, so the piece of bone was a couple of layers thick and using natural tissue is better than prosthetic pieces.
• Unwiring my jaw
• Two sets of injections into the scars on my face to help lighten the color. This doesn't sound that bad, but the areas of my face were sore, so this was excruciating.
• Removing my tracheotomy tube. It was interesting because the hole closed within 24 hours
• They cut the bone above my top set of teeth so they could move my whole set of top teeth forward
• A prosthetic implant was put under my left eye to raise it up
• My nose was partially fixed. When the ventilator tube was pulled from my nose, the feeding tube in my right nostril formed it. Because the

left side of my face next to my nose is about 1/3 of an inch lower than the other, the other side my nose could not be completely fixed. Still today, my left nostril is about 70% closed. I could get the inside cut out which would help me stop sniffing, but the benefit versus pain is something that I can't justify.

• A piece of my left ear was attached to the transition between my left eye socket and left cheekbone because there was a jagged edge where the bone shattered.

• Part of my right eyelid was removed and attached to the outside of my left eye so it could temporarily be closed to allow the muscles to strengthen

• Part of my hard palate was cut out and sewn to my lower gum to save a tooth and it was required by the orthodontist before I could get braces

• Braces for 9 months. I wanted to get my braces finished quick, so rather than going in every 2 months and getting a slight adjustment, I went in every month and had the orthodontist do as much of an adjustment as he could, regardless of the pain.

• 3 root canals. When your teeth slam together, it will often kill nerves and down the road there will be a need for root canals.

• 6 minor surgeries to gradually open my left eye

• A piece of skin from my loin was transferred under my eye in attempt to give me the appearance of a cheekbone. With hindsight, this was not the solution and the doctor who said he did reconstructive surgery actually did a lot more cosmetic surgery.

• My left eyebrow was moved up. This procedure was unnecessary. The doctor just wanted to make money and this is important to watch out for. The best thing you want to hear from a doctor is that they are not qualified to do a surgery or that it is not necessary. This shows that they care more about you than their bank account.

• Revision of scars and removal of pavement

• Cartilage from my right ear was placed under the skin on the left side of my nose to give the appearance of a normal transition.

• 2 revisions to my tracheotomy scar so the scar did not move as much when I swallowed.

• Two small liposuction procedures to get enough fat to fill in the sunken area under my left eye and to give me the appearance of a cheekbone. When there is blunt trauma, there is some loss of the soft tissue and it can be replaced with fat. This was a major step in making my face look normal.

- 4 times I had the fat injected into my face
- 6 times the doctor used Kenalog to try and reduce the fat in the bubble area where the piece of my loin was removed from my left cheekbone because the fat kept filling the area
- Laser treatment to the bubble area on my left cheekbone to tighten up the skin and make it flat
- 18 crowns and 6 veneers so my teeth would contact better
- 4 sessions of laser treatment to remove the redness from where the bubble was on my left cheekbone

That is only a partial list. The thing to note here is that serious injuries are not fixed quickly and incremental procedures are often necessary. There was obviously an extraordinary amount of pain, but I somehow forged on. Although there still are things that could be fixed, they are simply not worth the pain. If I don't tell someone what happened, they only notice a slight red mark on my left cheekbone and my sniffing because my left nostril is partially closed.

Moving to Austin

It was time for me to move out of Colorado Springs. My friends had gone in a different direction, the city was filled with too many bad memories, and Colorado Springs was not large enough to have enough professional opportunities in sales that I wanted. So, I decided to take a chance and took a friend's recommendation to move to Austin, Texas.

I sorted through my belongings, gave a lot away, stored the rest, and packed some clothes, a few books, my computer and I was on the road. I had never been to Texas and people thought that it was strange for me to move down there because Texas does not have a good reputation in Colorado.

Once I arrived in Austin, I recognized that the city seemed to have a lot of potential for me. I stayed in a hotel where I set up my computer and started looking for jobs. Being in a new city when you are not working or going to school made it difficult to meet people. There was a lot of time alone and my depression increased to the point where I would try and sleep to escape the depression.

My stay in a hotel lasted only five weeks before I was hired to work in the Silicon Valley. After five weeks in Austin, I did not want to leave because I had fallen in love with the city. However, I needed to start working, so I was shortly on the road to the Silicon Valley.

Moving to the Silicon Valley

My experience in the Silicon Valley has a number of lessons. First, I was still having issues because of not being on the correct medicine. The two issues that made working very difficult were my confusion and anxiety.

Although I went to a highly rated doctor for brain injuries, my mental issues did not improve. At times, the switching of my medication actually made my mental state worse and before I left the Silicon Valley, my level confusion was high. Granted, over time my doctor probably would have found the right combination, but I did not have the time.

Let me take this chance to make a couple of observations. First, it takes time to find the right mix of medicines and the proper dosages. Although it is important to try normal things like working, it can also bring a lot of stress, disappointment, and depression when you are not able to perform like you used to at work.

Next, brain trauma changes your mental makeup so medicines will not have the same affect as they would with a person who has not experienced brain trauma. In addition, the dosage that a person with a brain injury would take is different than a person without a brain injury.

Third, the difference in quality of life is dependent on the psychiatrists and/or neurologist's ability to get a person on the right type, dosage, and mix of medications. So ask questions about what the doctor specializes in, tell them how you feel, and it might even help to write down how you feel each day and at different times during the day.

I learned another lesson with a plastic surgeon. I found a plastic surgeon that told me he did a lot of reconstructive surgery and who had impressive medical training. Ultimately, he made some recommendations that, with hindsight, I see one procedure that was unnecessary and another that his solution did not address the cause of a problem. This was the doctor who moved my eyebrow when it was not necessary and who transferred the skin from my loin to my left cheekbone (not a good solution).

Even though I asked this plastic surgeon questions and my maxillofacial from Colorado Springs (Dr. Dombrowski) spoke with him before the surgery to make sure he had a good plan, the surgery ended up yielding poor results. I believe that this was pretty much all that I could do to check out a doctor, but watch out, because not all doctors have your best interest at heart and many think that they are capable of procedures when they are not.

The third item was that jumping to a new city, just like going to Austin, which is challenging in general and when you are having mental issues it becomes extremely challenging. With one of the hallmarks of head trauma being depression, not knowing anyone and being alone will really increase levels of depression. If you need to leave your city, just be prepared.

Although I had other job offers on the table, I was not happy in the Silicon Valley and in June 2001 (two years and three months after the accident) I decided to move back to Austin.

Moving Back to Austin

Within twenty-four hours of my decision, I packed up my clothes, computer and some other items into my Four-Runner, dropped off everything else at Goodwill, and I was back on the road to Austin.

Although I knew from the 5 weeks that I was in Austin before that I would be alone which would cause depression, there were no other options. I saw Austin as potentially a great place to live, I did not like the Silicon Valley, and the other locations were not feasible options, so it was going to be a struggle that I knew I had to face.

After driving and sleeping in my vehicle, I finally reached Austin and was happy because it was the right choice and a new beginning. I checked into an extended stay hotel, got my computer set up, and the process of building a new life in Austin started. The happiness quickly faded because this was just another place to be alone and to have confusion, depression, and anxiety.

Although it is my subjective observation, again, it is difficult when you alone in a new city to build a social network. If you have one friend or a girlfriend, it seems easier to me to start building relationships. This is especially true when you do not work, so you don't have co-workers to build relationships or when you are not in school, so you do not have fellow students to start a social network.

My father reiterated on a regular basis to find something that I liked to do even if it was not working. Ultimately, he knew that finding things for me to get up for and enjoy would help my depression, which could help my confusion, and might possibly get me back into a normal life.

The only two things that I liked to do were to play softball and to run. I eventually found an outdoor social group that had an extremely poor softball team, but it was a weekly event and it got me out of the hotel. Running was another activity that I could look forward to on a daily basis that got me out of the hotel, which had quickly become very depressing to be in.

I utilized a dating site to meet new people which ended up working after a few months when I met two girls who were looking to expand their social network. Even today, 7 years later, we are all still close friends.

The next phase was to find a new group of doctors and I lucked out and found two amazing doctors that eventually changed my life in an extremely positive ways. The first was a practicing neurologist who was also a practicing psychiatrist who was a perfect match for my situation. My depression, confusion, and anxiety at this point in June of 2001 (two years and three months after my accident) were as bad as ever.

Over the next couple of months, my mental issues had improved. I think neurologically after six months of seeing my new doctor that the medicine was as good as we could get it, but the remaining depression was based more on my situation in life.

The second doctor, Dr. John Jones, was the first maxillofacial or plastic surgeon who had the solution of injecting fat into areas of my face to fix my inset looking left eye and also a solution to give me the appearance of having a cheekbone. Facial deformity is brutal to deal with. Not only do you not look the same as you did before, but the big issue is that you look deformed.

After hearing Dr. Jones solution, I did have some hope to be able to "swallow the accident." By this I mean that at some point you become satisfied with the way that you look and you can move on with your life. Fixing my left eye and left cheekbone in addition to a number of other non-physical items was necessary to "swallow the accident."

After the first two surgeries people who did not know that I was in an accident would not have known by looking at me. After surgery doctor Jones, as well as other doctors, told me to look close at my face multiple times daily to make sure that there was not any infection.

The downside of this was that I became too critical of minor things that no one would ever notice. Even after I really did look normal, I still pushed for more changes, but Dr. Jones told me that I did not need those changes. This, as noted before, is very good news because when a doctor tells you that you should not get more surgery, you know that you have found a good doctor who has your best interest at heart over his/her bank account.

Eliminating the facial deformity was a gigantic milestone, but there were still a number of items mentally, socially, and professionally that would need to come together before I could honestly put the accident behind me.

Going Back to School

The Y2K technology build up, dot-com crash, other businesses going under, and finally 9-11 made the job market tough. Additionally, I was tired of working for other companies. I knew that I needed to get out of sales because of the stress and long hours, and to accomplish this, I decided to go back to school.

I wanted to start my own business, but I choose accounting and finance as my major so I would have a back up if I could not figure out a business to start or if my business went under.

This was kind of a last roll of the dice to recover mentally and professionally. I knew that if I failed, my depression would get to a critical level, and I would be out of options. It was time to try something because part of my depression was that I had nothing to get up for in the morning, felt hopeless, and viewed the rest of my life as me being a failure and miserable.

I spoke with the Dean of the Graduate Business department at Texas State University who told me that because I already had a bachelor's degree, it would be better to enter the university as a graduate student, take my undergraduate prerequisites and then my graduate classes. I started studying for the entrance exam to graduate school and I was terrified that I would not do well enough to get into the graduate program, but between my good undergraduate g.p.a. and graduate entrance exam score, I was able to get in.

Because of my high level of motivation, I thought that I was going to be able to take large number of classes, but shortly after I started class, I recognized that this was not the case. It was not that I had not been in school for a number of years, but I found that I had to relearn a lot of things due to the head injury and because I still had confusion.

My first semester started in January of 2002, which I was happy about the possibility of a new beginning, but scared because of failing at school. Actually the word "terrified" more aptly described how I felt.

To be able to learn and remember the material, I had to study for eighty hours a week while only taking four freshmen level business courses. My math, logic and critical thinking, memory, and writing skills were all very poor due to my brain injury which necessitated my need to study so many hours per week.

I decided that I needed to do everything possible to be successful in school, which included very intuitive things, but things that most students do not do. For instance my plan included reading the material to be discussed before class, trying some of the practice problems before class, re-writing my notes after class, re-reading the chapter discussed after class, and trying the problems over.

When I did not get a problem correct, I would go back and re-read that section and try that problem over or try a similar problem. I purchased the study guides to have more practice and wrote down important material and equations on note cards so whenever I was not in class or studying I could review them. I also asked professors' a lot of questions.

On the first few tests I was able to get in the 80th percentile which looking back was amazing, but I had always been able to be in the 90th percentile, so I studied even harder. The second round of tests I was able to get in the 90th percentile and I was able to achieve a 4.0 that end of my first semester.

With good grades, letters of recommendations from my professors and a convincing letter, I was awarded a Graduate Merit Scholarship. I went spring, summer and fall for two years for a total of 6 semesters. My ending g.p.a. was 3.94, so my success had continued. Although the amount of hours I had to study was less in the later semesters, I still studied a lot more than the other students in my classes.

December 2003 was my last semester. I had not graduated, but gained an impressive amount of knowledge and because I found a business I could start on my own, I left school.

Starting My Own Business

I started a business selling motorcycle related t-shirts online and went to a limited number of motorcycle rallies to sell shirts. To be able to get online sales without spending money on advertising or pay per click advertising (money that I did not have), I had to learn how to get my site on top of search engine results naturally.

This entailed learning search engine optimization (SEO). For people who grew up when computers were popular and when there were classes on computers starting in elementary school, it would be easier for them to learn SEO than for me because I did not grow up in that era.

Not only would I have to learn search engine optimization, but I would also have to learn how to write computer code. A partner and I found a search engine optimization company that, for a reasonable fee, showed me how to do both.

Eventually, I recognized that having money in inventory was not what I wanted. Also, for me to be successful selling shirts I would need a lot more money that I did not have to expand my offering and go to rallies full time which my limited bank account and back could not handle.

So I phased the shirts out and started focusing on providing rally information. The SEO company consultant had told me that it was important to have a lot of pages to be able to get visitors for a lot of different phrases. I had selected rally information because it was hard to find the information at the time and this ended up being a great choice.

After sixteen months of working on learning SEO and computer code between a limited number of rallies, I was getting enough traffic to start selling advertising.

Selling Advertising and Consulting

It was in the beginning of 2005 (about six years after the car accident) when I started selling advertising. In approximately nine months, I was able to secure enough advertisers to cover my basic living expenses.

While selling advertising, people started asking how I got so much traffic to my site and if I could help their site get more traffic. So, I started optimizing other companies' websites. Basically, I stumbled into another way to generate money.

While optimizing other companies' websites, the owners started asking me other questions about their site's layout and graphics, products that they should carry, rallies that were profitable to attend, basic business questions, marketing strategies, and more. So now, I was not only generating money from advertising and optimizing, but also consulting.

Eventually, I was making companies hugely successful and I was only charging a one-time fee for the optimization and consulting. For new clients, I decided that the only way that I would work with them was if I got a percentage of the business. I was able to work this deal with a few different companies and it has worked out well.

The cool thing that I recognized is that every six months or so, I could look back and see that the quality of these companies improved. Some of the early companies that I worked with where not set up to be successful, for instance, they did not have the money to buy enough products or to execute the marketing plan. With those companies, we negotiated a fair deal for both parties involved for me to end my work with them.

Toward the end of 2006 (seven and a half years after the accident), an inventor who had the biggest inventions in the motor sports industry since the motorcycle helmet contacted me. I was given 50% of the net profit to make the inventions successful in the market, which was simply huge.

Life Coming Together

On the eighth anniversary of my car accident, March 21, 2007, my struggle was complete. My face and physical issues were at a level that I was happy with, mentally and emotionally I was doing good, I was on the right medicine, found many close friends, had success in college, was professionally successful, and financially successful which allowed me to be at peace. Actually, it was a step further; I was content and I would not change anything in my life and did not need nor want anything else.

Though many of my successes were because of my motivation, I was also fortunate and blessed to have not destroyed parts of my brain. I was lucky to have the support of family and friends, and extremely lucky to have my father's love, friendship, encouragement, and support.

Although it took eight years, I was able to make a comeback that no one ever would have thought possible. Whether there is only potential for a partial recovery or a full recovery; there is hope.

LaVergne, TN USA
17 December 2010
209209LV00002B/88/P